HEALTHY SNACKS FOR KIDS

Quick & Nutrition Rich Snacks for Kids – Ideas With Their Recipes

By

JOHN GRAY

Table of contents

Introduction

Children can be fastidious eaters and get exhausted rapidly. With school life, nurturing, schoolwork burdens, and a ton of chaotic tomfoolery, the last thing you need to ponder is what to prepare for their lunch.

Snacks nowadays on the basic food item passageway are loaded with added sugars, carbs, and bunches of additives and secret fixings. We accept great nourishment starts with making snacks utilizing clean fixings. Your children shouldn't think twice about their wellbeing while at the same time partaking in their number one bites and neither would it be a good idea for you.

Assuming you are attempting to add more nutrients, minerals, and fiber to your kid's eating routine, then, at that point, these bites will cover your bases. Best of all, they never get exhausted and are totally heavenly. A portion of these tidbits are likewise without gluten and veggie lovers which implies your children won't be experiencing food sensitivities or any responsive qualities. We want to believe that you partake in the rundown.

Low-carb Little Zucchini Pizzas

In the event that you're searching for low-carb snacks for your children, this one will fulfill your necessities. The pizza sauce in addition to the fixings make it super scrumptious.

Smaller than expected Zucchini Pizzas

Fixings

Zucchini - One enormous (cut corner to corner in ¼ cuts)
Salt - 1/8 tsp
Pepper - 1/8 tsp
Pizza sauce - 1/3 cup
Mozzarella cheddar - ¾ cup
Smaller than expected pepperoni cuts - ½ cup
New basil leaves (cleaved)
Absolute Time

20 minutes

24 servings

Technique

Oil a baking sheet and preheat your kettle. Make the zucchini cuts fresh by cooking them

3 to 4 inches away from the barbecue for 1 to 2 minutes.

Add salt, pepper, pizza sauce, and the pepperoni cuts on top. Cook until the cheddar dissolves for about one more moment. Decorate with hacked basil leaves and serve hot.

Peanut Butter And Jam Apples

Peanut Butter and Jam sandwiches are a #1 among kids? In any case, what might be said about the people who are on sans gluten and eat less? The response is - Peanut Butter And Jam Apples!

Fixings

New apples - Two entirety
Simmered peanut butter - ¼ cup
Jam - ¼ cup
All out Time

10 minutes

4 servings

Technique

Make ¼-inch cuts longitudinally for the apples.
Utilize a cutout to make a cut at the center close to the middle.
Spread the peanut butter between the cuts and layer them like how you would make a sandwich.

Pour Jam through the middle center you recently made and you are finished.

Monster Trail Blend Munchies

These monster Trail Blend Munchies are a phenomenal treat for any individual who needs to partake in the decency of oats and Peanut butter. Your children will adore it!

Fixings

Exemplary moved oats - 1 cup
Small chocolate chips - ½ cup
Hacked peanuts - ¼ cup
Raisins - ¼ cup
Small M and Ms - ¼ cup
Smooth peanut butter - ¾ cup
Honey - 1 tbsp
Genuine salt
Absolute Time

30 minutes

12 servings

Technique

Snatch an enormous bowl and mix in the oats, chocolate chips, scaled down M and Ms, peanut butter, and honey.

Season this mix with salt and make small balls out of it by emptying them into tablespoons.

Refrigerate for 1-2 hours until these balls solidify and serve.

Peach Crumble Treat

Kids love peaches which is the reason we thought adding this pastry as a section would make their days much better. Fortunately it's truly sound and you'll adore it as well!

Fixings

Ready Peaches (Stripped and cut) - 6 cups
Earthy colored sugar - ¼ cup
Regular baking flour - 3 tbsp
Lemon juice - 1 tsp
Ground Lemon Zing - ½ tsp
Ground cinnamon - ½ tsp
For the garnishes:

Regular baking flour - 1 cup
Sugar - 1 cup
Baking powder - 1 tsp
Salt - ¼ tsp
Ground nutmeg - ¼ tsp
Egg - 1 enormous
Margarine - ½ cup (softened)
Vanilla frozen yogurt (discretionary)
All out Time

50 minutes

12 servings

Technique

Preheat the broiler to 375 degrees and put the peaches on a lubed sheet on the stove. Get a little bowl and in it blend earthy colored sugar, flour, lemon zing, and cinnamon.

Sprinkle peaches on the bowl and mix in flour, sugar, baking powder, salt, and nutmeg. Mix until the blend seems to be a brittle surface. Once more, sprinkle peaches and add margarine over the fixing.

Prepare the blend on the stove for around 40 minutes and top the sweet with cold vanilla frozen yogurt.

Banana Sushi

Bananas transformed into sushi, besides without the rice. We can read your mind however trust us, it's a sound tidbit!

Fixings

Ready banana - 1 entire (stripped)
Peanut butter - 2 tablespoons (softened)
Slashed strawberries - 2 tbsp
Scaled down chocolate chips - 2 tbsp
Squashed Graham saltines - 2 tbsp
All out Time

10 minutes

2 servings

Technique

Cut the bananas such that it seems to be sushi cuts.
Shower the liquefied peanut butter on it.
Top the cuts with the cleaved strawberries, small chocolate chips, and crushed Graham wafers.
Serve right away.

Mexican Firm Chickpeas

Skirt the chips and cheddar wafers for snacks by preparing these scrumptious however tasty Mexican Fresh Chickpeas. You will not be let down.

Mexican Firm Chickpeas

Fixings

Chickpeas - One 15-ounce can
Olive Oil - 1 tbsp
Legitimate salt
For the seasoning:

Cumin Powder - 1 tsp (grounded)
Coriander powder - 1 tsp (grounded)
Lemon zing - 1 tsp (grounded)
Complete Time

40 minutes

6 servings

Technique

Preheat the stove to 475 degrees and wipe off the chickpeas in the wake of eliminating from

the can. Ensure the skins are eliminated and put them on an oiled baking sheet. Shower olive oil, salt, and dish the chickpeas until they turn fresh which ought to require around 40 minutes.
Add the flavoring, let it cool a little, and serve.

Cooked Apples with Yogurt

Assuming that your children disdain apples, you can alter their perspectives with this basic yet sound recipe. These make for extraordinary school snacks.

Fixings

New apples - Two entire (cut up and cored)
Olive oil - 1 tbsp
Thyme - 4 twigs
Vanilla Greek yogurt
Absolute Time

20 minutes

2 servings

Technique

Cut up the apples on their sides and oil a baking sheet. Preheat your broiler, put the apples inside on the sheet, sprinkle with olive oil, and dish until they turn fresh. It ought to require around 20 minutes.

Add a touch of vanilla greek yogurt on top, decorate with a couple of twigs of thyme leaves, and serve.

Fox Toast

The Fox Toast is a delicious treat for even the fussiest of eaters. It's basically compelling and one of the most incredible Halloween snacks for youngsters.

Fox Toast

Fixings

Entire wheat bread - 4 cuts
Honey - 1 tbsp
Whipped cream cheddar - 1 cup
Rich peanut butter - 1 cup
Ready banana - 1 entire (cut)
Chocolate chips - 8 computers
New strawberries - 8 cuts
Blueberries - 4 entirety
Almonds - 8 cuts
Absolute Time

10 minutes

4 servings

Technique

Blend the cream cheddar and honey in a bowl. Spread it over the lower part of the toast however leave a V-hole close to the top community.

Fill the remainder of the toast with smooth peanut butter. Top the toast with two banana cuts for the eyes. Add chocolate chips to the banana cuts for the eye spots.

Add a blueberry only underneath for the nose and the cuts of almonds over the eyes for the eyebrows.

For the fox ears, add the cut strawberries simply over the almond cuts.

Apple Cinnamon Organic product Roll Ups

Organic product Roll Ups have made young lives paramount yet these Apple Cinnamon Organic product roll ups make new young lives significantly more so. They are additionally great without gluten snacks.

Fixings

Granny Smith Apples - 4 huge ones (stripped and cleaved).
Water - 1/3 cup
Granulated sugar - 2 tbsp
Newly pressed lemon juice - 1 tbsp
Grounded cinnamon powder - 1 tsp
Complete Time

3 hours 20 minutes

4 to 6 servings

Technique

Preheat the broiler to 175 degrees Celsius. Line up a baking sheet and oil it with olive oil.

On a medium pan, blend the apples, lemon juice, cinnamon powder, sugar, and water. Heat to the point of boiling and stew until the fluid dissipates (ought to take 15 mins).

Mix this combination in a food processor and mix until you get a smooth surface.

Move to the baking sheet and heat for 3 to 4 hours until it's not any more tacky yet dry.

Utilize a paring blade to cut the blend in lengthy vertical stripes and serve.

Peanut Butter Apple Nachos

Peanut butter Apple Nachos are totally delectable. Your children will fall head over heels for this tidbit, ensured! They additionally work perfectly as snacks for youngsters parties on birthday events and exceptional events.

Fixings

New Granny Smith apples - 2 entire (cored and cut into wedge shapes)
Regular peanut butter - ¼ cup (warm and dissolved)
Granola - 2 tbsp
Dried cranberries - 1 tbsp
Absolute Time

5 minutes

2 servings

Technique

Get a serving plate.
Organize the apple wedges, shower the peanut butter on them, top with granola and cranberries, and serve right away.

Broccoli Bread With Cheddar

Assuming that your children disdain broccoli and are dependent on garlic bread, you can in any case assist them with adjusting their perspectives. This Broccoli Bread with Cheddar comes exceptionally near the genuine article and makes for a wonderful treat! Simply attempt it.

Fixings

New broccoli - 3 cups (pieces)
Entire egg - 1 huge
Destroyed Mozzarella Cheddar - 1 and ½ cup
Newly ground Parmesan - ¼ cup
Garlic cloves - 2 entire (minced)
Dried oregano - ½ tsp
Legitimate salt
Newly ground dark pepper
Crushed red pepper chips (squeezed)
Newly hacked parsley leaves - 2 tsp
Warmed marinara sauce (for serving)
Complete Time

40 minutes

8 servings

Technique

Preheat the stove to 425 degrees. Line up a baking sheet with material paper and oil it with olive oil. Put the diced broccoli in a bowl and microwave for 1 moment.

Get it out and utilize a cheesecloth to eliminate any overabundance dampness.

In a huge bowl, blend the riced broccoli now in with an egg, mozzarella cheddar, parmesan cheddar, and garlic. Blend oregano, salt, and pepper and use it for the flavoring.

Move the mixture to your baking sheet and shape it into a slender roundabout shape. Heat for around 20 minutes and shower it with ½ cup mozzarella cheddar. Heat for around 10 minutes until you get a liquefied mess outside that is likewise firm. Decorate with parsley and pepper pieces.

Serve hot with a smidgen of marinara sauce as an afterthought to oblige it.

Banana Penguins

Assuming your youngsters detest kid-accommodating vegetable tidbits, you can get them going no sweat your direction in. Furthermore, these Banana Penguins will precisely raise a ruckus around town.

Fixings

Bananas - 6 entirety
Liquefied chocolate - 1 cup
Liquefied coconut oil - 1 tbsp
Candy eyes - 24 pieces
Orange M&Ms - 36 computers
All out Time

35 minutes

12 servings

Technique

Eliminate the strips from the bananas and spot them in a little bowl. Top the backs and tips of the Bananas with dissolved chocolate.
Use treat eyes for making the eyes and make specks utilizing dissolved chocolate. Utilize a

touch of liquefied chocolate for the feet. Put orange M&Ms between the eyes for the nose and at the base to finish the feet.
Refrigerate and serve cold. Your Banana Penguins are fit to be eaten!

Apple Fries

Jump out the French fries and go with these Apple Fries all things being equal. Trust us, you'll cherish it, and besides, they are stacked with supplements.

Apple Fries

Fixings

Milk - ¾ cup
Egg - 1 enormous
Regular baking flour - 1 cup
Baking powder - 1 tsp
Sugar - 1/3 cup in addition to 2 tbsp (isolated)
Ground cinnamon powder - 3 ½ tsp
Vegetable Oil - 2 cups
Fit Salt - ¼ tsp
Granny Smith apples - 3 enormous ones (cored and stripped)
Warmed caramel sauce (for the plunge)
Absolute Time

25 minutes

12 servings

Technique

Get going by making the player for your Apple Fries. You do this by blending milk, egg, flour, baking powder, 2 tbsp sugar, ½ tsp cinnamon, and salt in a major blending bowl. Mix until there are no huge bunches.

Get a little bowl and blend 1/3 cup sugar with 3 tsp cinnamon powder for making the sprinkles or cleaning for the French fries.

Take a skillet and pour vegetable oil on it. Cut your apples into ½-inch wedges and dress them in the hitter.

Use cooking utensils to put the wedges in the oil and cook until they become brilliant brown. Rehash for the opposite side by flipping and cooking briefly.

Eliminate your broiled apples from the skillet and spot them in a plate fixed with paper towels. Channel the overabundance oil, sprinkle with the cinnamon-sugar tidying you made and serve.

Children's Birthday Popcorn

Children's birthday popcorn is a scrumptious wind to conventional birthday cakes. Your kids will need a greater amount of this whenever they're finished licking their lips.

Fixings

Light spread popcorn - 1 entire pack
White chocolate chips - 1 cup
Vegetable oil - 2 tbsp
Vanilla cake blend - 3 tbsp
Rainbow sprinkles - ¼ cup
All out Time

A couple of moments

1 serving

Technique

Open the light margarine popcorn sack and pop it in view of the guidelines given in the bundling.
Get a little, microwave-confirmation bowl and in it blend the vegetable oil in with white chocolate chips. Heat it in the microwave in

time periods seconds until they're both completely liquefied. Consolidate the vanilla cake blend and mix well.

Get a resealable pack (size ought to be of a gallon), put the popcorn in that alongside the vanilla cake and white chocolate chip blend. Leave out the bits, seal, and shake well until the popcorn is covered well and uniformly.

Design the popcorn on a different baking sheet and add sprinkles on top. Refrigerate for around 20 to 25 minutes and serve chilled.

Sans gluten Strawberry Oats Bars

Sans gluten Strawberry Cereal Bars give kids that economical energy without the sugar crash. They are a lot more grounded than your locally acquired cereal bars and they contain no troublesome fillers or additives. Also, the most awesome aspect? Your children can eat them faultlessly! We'll let you know the recipe.

Fixings

Coconut Oil - 4 tbsp (liquefied)
Non-fat Greek Yogurt - 2 tbsp
Egg - 1 entirety
Coconut sugar - 1/3 cup
Vanilla - 1 tsp
Himalayan Pink Salt - ¼ tsp
Baking pop - ½ tsp
Baking Powder - ¼ tsp
Cinnamon powder - ½ tsp
Ginger - ¼ tsp
Oat flour - 1 cup
Without gluten flour blend - ½ cup
Strawberry Jam - ¼ cup
Ground flaxseed dinner - 1 tbsp
Absolute Time

30 minutes

8 servings

Technique

Preheat the stove to 385 degrees Fahrenheit and line a baking sheet with material paper on it. Liquefy coconut oil in a microwave for around 30 seconds in a bowl and put away.
Get a little bowl and whisk Greek Yogurt and the egg. Join the coconut sugar, vanilla, cinnamon, ginger, baking pop, baking powder, and salt. Whisk well until it's smooth and there are no heating up powder bunches left.
Make the batter for the bars by including the oat flour, sans gluten flour blend, and coconut oil. Allow it to sit for 10 minutes and put away.
Get two sheets of wax paper and between them, carry out the mixture in 10 X 12 squares. Utilize a baked good blade to cut the mixture into eight equivalent squares and keep the excess pieces left for sometime in the future.
Pour the strawberry jam through the focal point of these bars the long way. Leave a little hole on the sides so they don't wind up getting crunched. Seal up the openings by pushing and shutting in the batter with your hands.

Put the bars on the stove and prepare for around 15 minutes until they turn puffed upward and prepared. Top with the flaxseed feast and move to a cooling rack. Serve when they are at room temperature or store away in water/air proof holders for later utilization.

Conclusion

What's more, that is all there is to it! Partake in these recipes, let your children eat however much they might want and never need to stress over going past their calorific admission while they're busy. As a matter of fact, with these bites, they will feel phenomenal truly as well as intellectually as well. Have a great time!

www.ingramcontent.com/pod-product-compliance
Lightning Source LLC
LaVergne TN
LVHW020535160826
845677LV00015B/4078

9798849603841